Physics of Consciousness

15 Ways Information and Energy are the Formula for all the Forces in the Universe

"Spirituality is an incomplete picture of reality without quantum physics."
~The Dalai Lama

Every moment of every day, your life is a blank canvas of creative unbounded possibilities. The powerful information within this book is an offering, an invitation for you to explore the quantum by tapping into higher levels of cosmic intelligence, universal consciousness.

This informative book:

- Explains how you are directing the unseen cosmic forces inside the body and the unseen cosmic forcers outside the body.
- Explores energies of the Pineal gland's gateway to enlightenment, DNA, qualia, string theory, energy, frequency and vibration and the quantum field.

Physics of Consciousness is exciting. Pick up your copy and begin to change your life today.

Your Amazing Itty Bitty® Physics of Consciousness Book

15 Quantum Events Shaking the World of Science to the Core

Rhona Jordan

C.GIt., C.CHt.

Published by Itty Bitty® Publishing
A subsidiary of S & P Productions, Inc.

Printed in the United States of America

Itty Bitty Publishing
311 Main Street, Suite D
El Segundo, CA 90245
(310) 640-8885

ISBN: 978-1-950326-36-5

Photograph of Rhona Jordan courtesy of Prasad Photographer.

Dedication

To my extraordinary grandchildren: Jordan, Ryan and Lauren.

Consciousness is like space in the sky, and your conscious thoughts and actions are the energy – the weather passing through. Your consciousness is here because you are to help change history during this pivotal time, you have a divine purpose. Each of you has special gifts and abilities. I am proud of you and love you beyond the quantum.

Stop by our Itty Bitty® website to find more information about the physics of consciousness at:

www.ittybittypublishing.com

Or visit Rhona Jordan at

www.RhonaImagery.com

Table of Contents

Quantum Event 1.	Definition of Consciousness
Quantum Event 2.	Panpstychism Science
Quantum Event 3.	Quantum Junction Points
Quantum Event 4.	Creation Began
Quantum Event 5.	Divine Design
Quantum Event 6.	DNA Consciousness
Quantum Event 7.	Pineal Gland Consciousness
Quantum Event 8.	Vibration Matches Potential
Quantum Event 9.	String Theory Changes Science
Quantum Event 10.	Consciousness in Everything
Quantum Event 11.	The Field
Quantum Event 12.	Quantum Entanglement
Quantum Event 13.	The Eye of Horus Grid
Quantum Event 14.	Qualia Science
Quantum Event 15.	Qualia Action for Quantum Success

Introduction

Physics of Consciousness

"Spirituality is an incomplete picture of reality without quantum physics."
~The Dalai Lama

Every moment of every day, your life is a blank canvas of creative unbounded possibilities and the powerful information within this book is an offering, an invitation for you to explore the quantum by tapping into higher levels of cosmic intelligence, universal consciousness.

This informative book explains how you are directing the unseen cosmic forces inside the body and the unseen cosmic forcers outside the body. We explore energies of the Pineal gland's gateway to enlightenment, DNA, qualia, string theory, energy, frequency and more.

Confucius said it best:

"Every thought you think is generating your future.
"Every act you do is cultivating your future.
"Every word you speak is creating your future.
"You must become aware of the thought that you are tossing out into the universe."

Quantum Event 1
Definition of Consciousness

In order to change a situation, biological organisms approach a situation and are able to change their behavior. They are conscious.

1. In each different state of consciousness, you have many different biological changes, awareness and perceptions.
2. Each state of consciousness offers vastly different experiences and knowledge.
3. When you are aware and observing your thoughts, consciousness from higher states are activated.
4. The ancient wisdom seers of the Vedanta Science in India taught about the seven states of consciousness. Each state of consciousness leads to another state and the states merge into each other.
5. Scientists are now beginning to think the universe is conscious.

States of Consciousness

- **1st State - Awake**: You are aware of activity and experiencing the five senses as real.
- **2nd State - Deep Sleep**: There is little awareness, desiring nothing and having no dreams.
- **3rd State - Dreaming**: All experiences in this reality feel real.
- **4th State - Transcendental**: Here you are glimpsing the soul, tapping into the cosmic state.
- **5th State - Cosmic**: You are the detached observer of your own body as if watching it from the outside, while the body is experiencing being awake, deep sleep, and dreaming.
- **6th State - Divine, God Consciousness**: The Soul is fully awake and sees everything as singular consciousness; there is no separation.
- **7th State - The Silent Ever-present Witness**: You know you are the entire ocean in the drop, not just a drop in the ocean; infinite love, freedom, liberation.

Quantum Event 2
Panpstychism Science
Shaking the World of Science to its Core

According to Albert Einstein, the words light or energy are the same, they are interchangeable.

1. Science: You are made of energy and everything in the universe is made of energy.
2. Science: In physics, a quantum (plural: quanta) is the minimum amount of any physical entity involved in an interaction.
3. Science: On the quantum physic level your thoughts and intentions become the particle or the wave of creation.
4. Science: You are made up of electron fluctuations that are popping in and out of existence.
5. Science: Every atom passing through your body is made up of the same components of a collapsed star. You are made of star dust.
6. Science: You are a conscious being and like the atom, consciousness is explosive with creative forces.
7. Scientists continue searching the mysteries to the universal questions of existence: why, when and how.

Quantum Vision Imagery

- Imagine you are the universe, the reality is you are. The quantum changes energy into matter and matter into energy.
- Observation affects the outcome; we aren't merely participants of the universe but participants in it.
- You and the universe are co-creator and director of self-fulfilling prophesy.
- Desire, like the atom is explosive with creative forces in the present moment when all possibilities exist in the quantum field, potentials become reality.
- Imagine you are a quantum physicist looking into the body through a microscope.
- Notice you are observing only a void, with energy packets of information appearing and disappearing.
- Imagine the intelligent energy influencing the biochemistry.
- Imagine shifting the energy of expanded awareness for healing. Imagine the calmed nervous system as patterns of light. Imagine balancing blood flow and blood chemistry. Imagine enhancing oxygen and nutrition molecules.
- Imagine you directing and shifting molecules of emotion. Imagine all the rhythms of the body as harmonious.
- Quantum direction is powerful.

Quantum Event 3
Quantum Junction Points

The body has quantum junction points for consciousness called chakras that communicate with the body distributing life force energy and information. Every living cell is affected by the color spectrum and the sound frequency of the quantum chakra. Quanta, energy, frequency, information are referred to as light. Once you know the chakra location, you can re-calibrate the quantum energy with meditation, yoga and imagination and intention.

Location of quantum junction points:

1. **First Chakra**: base of the tailbone
2. **Second Chakra**: spleen area, below the navel
3. **Third Chakra**: 2 inches above the navel
4. **Fourth Chakra**: center of the chest
5. **Fifth Chakra**: throat
6. Sixth **Chakra**: between the eyebrows (3rd eye)
7. **Seventh Chakra**: crown of the head
8. **Eighth Chakra**: 16 inches above the crown of the head

Imagery for Calibrating Quantum Junction Points

- **First Chakra** - Imagine connecting with earth energy and pulling the earth light up through your feet to the first chakra below the tailbone; color is red, hearing and feeling the sound vibration of "LAM".
- **Second Chakra** - Imagine pulling the light up to the spleen area; color is orange, hearing and feeling the sound vibration of "VAM".
- **Third Chakra** - Imagine pulling the light up 2 inches passed the navel; color is yellow, hearing and feeling the sound vibration of "RAM".
- **Fourth Chakra** - Imagine pulling the light up to the chest; color is green, hearing and feeling the sound vibration of "YUM".
- **Fifth Chakra** - Imagine pulling the light up to the throat; color is blue, hearing and feeling the sound vibration of "HUM".
- **Sixth Chakra** - Imagine pulling the light up to the third eye, color is indigo, hearing and feeling the sound vibration of "SHAM".
- **Seventh Chakra** - Imagine pulling the light up to the crown, color is violet, hearing and feeling the sound vibration "OM".

Quantum Event 4
Creation Began

The human nervous system, the brain, the mind is a manifesting quantum universe within you to become self-aware beyond the ego encapsulated identity.

1. We are not even close to fully understanding the complex brain, mind and their mysteries.
2. There is a multidimensional universe hiding inside our brain.
3. The Algebraic Topology computer programed with a virtual brain shows a combination of multi-dimensional geometrical structures and spaces.
4. In just a speck of the brain are tens of millions of multi-dimensional structures that can go up to eleven dimensions.
5. The higher dimensions are mathematical and are outside the realm of physics.
6. The quantum mind's thoughts can move molecules, change body chemistry.
7. The quantum mind can transcend into higher realms of consciousness.

The Human Nervous System

The body wants to be well and knows how to heal itself.

- Our thoughts and fears can get in the way of our inner intelligence either compromising the immune system and the nervous system or supporting health in these systems.
- In the Vedic teachings it says, "I am the universe" a higher state of being.
- The body is the great master teacher. It can bring you to your knees. When you learn to heal the body, you have learned about the cosmos.
- As above, so below. All is consciousness.
- Perceptions can create boundaries and rule your life or set it free.

Quantum Event 5
Divine Design
The Cosmic Mind with Devine Design
Creates the Self-Aware Universe

No one knows why or how:

1. The planets are traveling in perfect patterns, distance, rotation, movement, speed and creating amazing sacred geometric patterns when they are tracked.
2. Earth is 4.57 billion years old.
3. The third planet from the Sun is Earth.
4. 71 % of the Earth is covered by water.
5. The Earth's core is liquid with a solid inner center; the inner core rotates slightly faster than the rest of the planet.
6. Earth's magnetic field is caused from the outer iron rich core combined with the energy of Earth's rotation.
7. Life appeared within one billion years of earth's formation.
8. The atmosphere we enjoy today began 2.7 billion years ago.
9. The speed of light is 670 million mph.
10. NASA records the sounds of planets from space. Earth's sound is "AUM".
11. Scientists are now pondering consciousness in the divine design of the universe.

Conscious Intelligence is Creating the Universe, the Planets and You

- Quanta, consciousness, meaning and intelligence play key roles.
- Consciousness is infinite creativity.
- Consciousness surrounds you and is within you.
- Consciousness is everywhere, the collective; consciousness is the in the flower, rock or bird looking back at you.
- Consciousness observes you and you observe it.
- Consciousness is the fundamental source of creation.
- Consciousness was first and then the Universe formed; consciousness was first and then you are formed.
- Consciousness is life and death, energy changing form.
- Consciousness' higher levels are expanded cosmic expression.
- Consciousness is inspired thought, creation and action.
- Consciousness is the field, the womb of creation, pure unbounded potentiality.
- Consciousness and all the universes expand together.
- Consciousness and you co-create together.

Quantum Event 6
DNA Consciousness

DNA (Deoxyribonucleic Acid) is the genetic geometry blueprint found in all living things. DNA has coded messages of expression that are greater in numbers than the subatomic particles in our solar system. That is a lot of consciousness.

1. Any one part of the DNA is a hologram of the whole.
2. DNA is a hologram of your consciousness.
3. Families are genetically interconnected through the DNA
4. Genetic inheritance results from the DNA's ability to duplicate itself in a self-replicating pattern.
5. Every living cell is made of just six elements: carbon, calcium, hydrogen, oxygen, phosphorus, and nitrogen.
6. DNA appears as a spiral ladder with a series of rungs holding together the two vertical strands on each side.
7. The DNA double helix requires ten rungs to make a complete spiral turn.
8. DNA combines into strands called chromosomes.
9. Humans have 46 Chromosomes (23 pairs).

More about DNA Consciousness

The DNA double helix is a 3-D spiral related to growth and Sacred Geometry. Its form can be seen in cyclones, hurricanes, honeysuckle, morning glory plants and the horns of an antelope or ram. The ancient Greeks created the Caduceus, a symbol for medicine with two serpents curled around a wand resembling the DNA structure long before the discovery of the spiral human DNA in 1953.

- DNA has the same mathematical formula: Pi, Golden Mean, Sacred Geometry.
- DNA is energy and frequency.
- All frequency carries information.
- DNA is consciousness.

Quantum Event 7
Pineal Gland Consciousness

The pineal gland is located deep in the brain. It looks like a tiny pinecone and is the size of a large grain of rice. It is the antenna for receiving elevated consciousness information. The properties of the pineal gland are:

1. It is piezoelectric; it experiences electric polarity.
2. Its calcite crystals are made of carbon, oxygen approximately 1 to 20 microns in length.
3. The pineal gland receives and converts signals.
4. It is a neuroendocrine transducer; it converts variations in a physical quantity into an electrical signal, or vice versa.
5. Like radio waves, or TV antenna, the pineal gland becomes a transducer, electrically activated and generates an electrometric field.
6. The pulsating pineal gland picks up the pulsating signal from the pulsating fields and converts the signal into meaningful information.
7. The pineal gland picks up electromagnetic frequencies that travel faster than the speed of light.

The Pineal Gland is called the Third Eye

When the pineal gland is activated, it:

- Picks up frequencies above our three-dimensional reality and expands awareness beyond the five senses.
- Picks up higher dimensions of consciousness.
- Connects with energy, frequency, and information from higher consciousness that become vivid imagery in the brain and mind.
- Heightens multisensory visions by releasing melatonin that is transmuted into profound chemical neurotransmitters in the brain as you are experiencing the transcendence experience.

Imagery
- Imagine the Eye of Horus grid lighting up the brain (see Quantum Event #13).
- Receive direct download frequency (information).
- Breathe in the sacred teachings.
- Channel higher awareness, higher consciousness.
- Connect with primordial awareness.
- Become one with all beings; one with the collective consciousness.
- Imagine pure light, transcendence.
- You are now in the field where there is no time, no space, nowhere, non-local.

Quantum Event 8
Vibration Matches Potential
Your State of Being

Words send out the electrical charge. Strong emotions send out the magnetic charge. The combined charges create the electromagnetic signature.

1. The electromagnetic signature is equal to your state of being.
2. You are pulling the equal state toward you.
3. You are directing molecules of emotions.
4. You are directing the quantum and its wave in the field of all possibility.
5. You are consciousness working with consciousness.
6. You are magnetic.

Imagery for Vibration and Potential

- Imagine the body as matter.
- Imagine the matter as energy.
- Image the energy activity of electrons popping in and out of the void and tiny fluctuating information packets flashing here and here and over there and there.
- Imagine being able to see millions of molecules spinning in space.
- Imagine influencing the invisible quantum forces.
- Imagine the intelligent energies of consciousness in the universal field.
- Imagine you are the co-creator with the universe.
- Imagine you are the director of your vision.
- Feel your vision, taste it, be it.
- Experience your vision as if it has already happened.
- You are the creator, the creation and the observer of the creation.
- Your imagination is powerful beyond measure.

Quantum Event 9
String Theory Changes Science
Consciousness Showing Its Self

String theory is a mathematical equation. String theory physicists are hoping to tie physics into one equation. It is one of the most unusual scientific theories of all time and has yielded many unexpected results.

1. String theory was first studied in 1968 and is still a work in progress.
2. It has driven major developments in mathematics and insights.
3. String theory is also part of quantum field theory, studying extra dimensions that provide geometric description of all the particles and forces known to modern physics.
4. No proven theory exists to explain the beginnings of our conscious life or the cosmic coincidences in universe.
5. String theory science may eventually prove that the universe and all that we know is consciousness, much like a vast plasma neural network, perhaps a cosmic mind.

Your Consciousness is Expanding with the Ever-expanding Universe

String theory & quantum field theory allow for:

- Wormholes to create shortcuts in our universe to distant parallel universes
- Time travel
- Hologram universe
- Multidimensional dimensions of time and space
- Black holes
- Space-time
- Life beyond Earth
- Galactic consciousness
- Quantum teleportation

Quantum Event 10
Consciousness in Everything

Consciousness is everywhere and in everything.

1. Some people have had the experience of hearing the moaning sounds made by trees as they are being burned or cut down.
2. Scientists have experimented with household plants. In one study, a leaf was cut and the scissors left near the plant. When the scientist returned and picked up the scissors the plant immediately registered activity on the computer readings.
3. A study by Japanese scientist, Dr. Massaru Emoto, is proving that words, thoughts and intentions can affect the environment. You can watch one of his experiments with rice on YouTube in which he treats rice placed in three different glass jars differently. He uses kind words toward jar #1, ugly words toward jar #2 and he ignores jar #3.
4. Dr. Emoto's experiment shows that at the end of the month, jar #1 fermented and smelled nicely, jar #2 turned black and jar #3 started to rot.

Tree Consciousness Imagery

- Journey inward, deep into the quantum world.
- Imagine the tree as energy, as light.
- Imagine the tree roots deep in the earth.
- Imagine the seasons, sun and clouds, wind and rain, heat and cold.
- Imagine the bird nest and squirrels in the tree.
- Imagine the conversation between you and the tree; the tree saying, "Give me your burdens and I will send them deep into the earth for transformation".
- Imagine the tree transferring strength, Earth wisdom and knowledge to you.
- Imagine feeling the bark on the side of your face as your body hugs the tree.
- Imagine the tree saying, "I can feel the blood running through your veins and you can feel the sap traveling in the center of my trunk. We are one being, one consciousness".

Quantum Event 11
The Field
AKA: Quantum Field, Unified Field,
Field of all Possibilities
Pure Consciousness

Definitions of the quantum field:

1. Pure unbounded potential
2. Pure possibility
3. Unbounded awareness
4. A cosmic realm beyond 3-dimensional reality
5. Enlightenment
6. Womb of creation
7. A unique expression of everything in existence
8. Pure energy changing form
9. No place
10. No time
11. No space
12. Nonlocal

To see a world in a grain of sand
And a heaven in a wild flower
Hold infinity in the palm of your hand
And eternity in an hour

- **William Blake**

William Blake's words stretch us far beyond our everyday perception and into the quantum. They represent his inner vision of unbounded awareness in the field of all possibilities.

- Your abilities are beyond measure in the field.
- Quantum field awareness promotes overall balance in mind/body.
- Increases resistance to lower frequencies and disease.
- Increases a sense of vibrant health, connectedness to a greater source.
- Self-directs biological transformation
- Every thought you have is already encoding a biological choice for directed energy that is creating balance or imbalance in the body.
- The vibrating cells change instantly as your thoughts direct your evolution.

Quantum Event 12
Quantum Entanglement

Quantum entanglement means that everything in the universe is connected in some way and on some level everywhere all the time.

1. The world of quantum physics shows that nothing is as it seems.
2. We are a collective consciousness and that is what is holding existence together.
3. The core of everything, including you, is made up of small particle building blocks of pure energy creating your reality.
4. The core of all existence is intertwined, entangled with energetic networks of pure information.
5. Quantum physics scientists know that depending on different circumstances, sub-atomic particles behave differently. Observation effects the way particles behave.
6. There is no scientific knowledge of why or how entanglement transmits information. Essentially, quantum entanglement suggests that acting on a particle here can instantly influence a particle far away and the implications are huge for quantum mechanics and quantum computing.

Spooky Action at a Distance

Dr. Albert Einstein called it "spooky action at a distance", meaning that two objects remain connected without communication in any conventional way through time and space, long after their initial interaction has taken place.

- Once particles have interacted, they remain connected, energetically entangled.
- No matter the physical distance, they remain affected by one another.
- Physical reality is a single quantum system that responds together.
- Photons, electrons, or any atomic object may be curiously entangled.
- How does the mind sometimes know who is calling before the phone rings?
- Collective consciousness is entanglement.
- Empty space, the quantum vacuum itself, may be filled with entangled particles, a deeply interconnected reality.

Quantum Event 13
The Eye of Horus Grid

If thine eye be single, thy whole body
shall be full of light.
~ Matthew 6.22

The Eye of Horus is the fractal grid superimposed on the brain by the formation and locations of the pineal gland, corpus callosum, hypothalamus, pituitary gland and thalamus. It is a symbol signifying power, health and protection used by the ancient Egyptians who practiced higher levels of consciousness. It is the entry into other realms of consciousness.

1. When the hypothalamus is stimulated it communicates with the pituitary gland secreting neurohormones.
2. The pituitary gland releases oxytocin, the love chemical, and vasopressin that retain fluids to carry greater frequencies of information that affect the thalamus.
3. The pineal gland contains crystals that when activated become the antenna picking up a higher frequency beyond sensory-based reality and transforms the information in the brain into vivid surreal images.

More about the Eye of Horus Grid

The fractal grid superimposed over the brain starting at the pineal gland shows that within the grid lays the pineal gland, thalamus, hypothalamus, corpus callosum, together creating the perfect formation of the Eye of Horus.

- The pineal gland is stimulated by the sound of "OM" vibrating in the skull, meditation, darkness, the tongue positioned towards the uvula, back of the mouth. Breath-work creates pressure that forces the flow of cerebrospinal fluid up the spine activating the Eye of Horus grid increasing energy, frequency, information, vibration, expanded awareness, higher levels of consciousness, enlightenment, dimensional travel beyond space and time.
- Hermes, holding a Caduceus, was a messenger of the gods. In Greek mythology, Hermes had the ability to enter different dimensions and other worlds. The Caduceus is a stick/rod with two snakes wrapped around it. Near the top are bird wings spread open as in flight. Just above the bird wings at the very top of the stick/rod is a pinecone, representing the pineal gland.

Quantum Event 14
Qualia Science

The word "qualia" is Latin for "qualities" toward subjective experience, the glue that holds the five senses together: light, sound, color, shape, and texture.

1. Every experience you have is made up of qualia (the glue).
2. The body is a bundle of qualia.
3. The brain's experiences are qualia.
4. Qualia become consciousness-based from the physical.
5. Dimensions in space-time, the four-dimensional continuum, contain qualia.
6. Pure consciousness is the source of qualia.
7. All subjective experiences are qualia such as: perception, cognition, love, compassion, suffering and pleasure.
8. Qualia are: insight, intuition, imagination, inspiration, creativity.

More about Qualia Science

The body is the experience of qualia: speech, mental activity, and interactions.

- Qualia are the senses and perceptions.
- Qualia are a feedback loop that originates in consciousness.
- Qualia register experiences in the brain.
- Qualia are the potential.
- We experience empathy through our shared qualia.
- The universe fits our perspective, our qualia.
- Qualia science is leading us to understand enlightenment.

Quantum Event 15
Qualia Action for Quantum Success
Qualia Vision Board

A proven, powerful approach to making your dreams a reality is to prepare a Qualia Vision Board. These are the tools you will need:

1. Poster board
2. Glue stick
3. Scissors
4. Photos
5. Colored markers or drawing tools
6. Written affirmations, meaningful words
7. A list of what you want
8. How would you feel when what you want is manifested?
9. Are you ready for these changes in your life?
10. Be very, very clear exactly what you want.
11. Set aside time to create the vision.
12. Prepare and gather your Qualia Vision Board tools.
13. Consider holding a vision board gathering with your friends for powerful group synergy and support.
14. Consider you and the children working on your vision boards around the kitchen table.

How to Make a Qualia Vision Board

- The universe says "tell me what you want. I am unbounded, unlimited, I am all possibilities, I am creation and you are the co-creator".
- Decide what you want: love, health, family, abundance, physical comforts, a vacation, to heal a relationship or create a new relationship, a different job, etc.
- Look at the blank poster board and feel the emotions of creating your desired future consciously.
- As you cut and glue pictures of your desires from magazines, photos or drawings, say out loud (electrical charge) in gratitude that you are thankful the event or thing has already happened.
- The universe is abundant and it is yours; feel strongly the emotion (magnetic charge). You are attracting the magnetically equal state of being to you.
- Beneath your pictures glue meaningful, powerful words and say the powerful affirmations/words out loud.
- Every day look at your Qualia Vision Board and affirm your intentions, celebrate your desires as if they have already come to you.
- You are working consciously with qualia, awareness and universal consciousness.
- Make your quanta vision grand.

You've finished. Before you go…

Tweet/share that you finished this book.

Please star rate this book.

Reviews are solid gold to writers. Please take a few minutes to give us some itty bitty feedback.

ABOUT THE AUTHOR

Rhona, an inquisitive Aquarian, is intrigued by the movement of the stars, awareness of day to day consciousness, levels of consciousness, the creation of the universe, the how, when, and why of existence.

Rhona's continued search for answers has led her to the scientific study of quantum physics, a field which has created more questions than answers. However, those answers have changed the world of science as we knew it and the way Rhona now shares global information.

Rhona uses the science of the quantum, awareness of consciousness and the power to create in all her offerings: mediation, imagery, clinical hypnosis, lectures, teaching classes, or helping patients prepare for a procedure.

Rhona shares her teaching of magnetics and energy by addressing the cells, molecules, atomic and sub atomic particles of the body's internal wisdom for change and wellbeing.

Rhonas has a private practice and her services are also offered in a major hospital and several clinics in Orange County, California. For more information, please refer to her website at: www.rhonaimagery.com or by email at: Rhonaimagery@aol.com

When you had that thought, creation began!

Other Amazing Itty Bitty Books

- **Your Amazing Itty Bitty® Imagery Book**
  – Rhona Jordan, C.GIt., C.CHt.

- **Your Amazing Itty Bitty® Meditation Book**
  – Rhona Jordan, C.GIt., C.CHt.

- **Your Amazing Itty Bitty® Interstitial Cystitis Book**
  – Rhona Jordan, C.GIt., C.CHt.

With many more Amazing Itty Bitty® books available online...